Carla Patricia Penelas da Costa

Evaluation of the incidence of occupational accidents in the veterinary field

Carla Patricia Penelas da Costa

Evaluation of the incidence of occupational accidents in the veterinary field

ScienciaScripts

Imprint

Cover image: www.ingimage.com

This book is a translation from the original published under ISBN 978-620-2-04109-6.

Publisher:
Sciencia Scripts
is a trademark of
Dodo Books Indian Ocean Ltd. and OmniScriptum S.R.L publishing group

120 High Road, East Finchley, London, N2 9ED, United Kingdom
Str. Armeneasca 28/1, office 1, Chisinau MD-2012, Republic of Moldova, Europe
Managing Directors: Ieva Konstantinova, Victoria Ursu
info@omniscriptum.com

Printed at: see last page
ISBN: 978-620-8-41352-1

EVALUATION OF THE INCIDENCE OF OCCUPATIONAL ACCIDENTS WITH POTENTIAL BIOLOGICAL HAZARDS AND IMPLEMENTING CORRECTIVE BEHAVIORAL MEASURES IN VETERINARY PROFESSIONALS

Today, we continue to see high levels of accidents, possibly reflecting poor or non-existent occupational risk prevention structures in many workplaces. The need for safety, hygiene, prevention and training at work is, at the same time, a reflection on ourselves and our attitudes as priority players, increasingly dependent and demanding on work and everything it entails.

However, workplaces often create dangerous situations for workers' health and physical integrity. Worldwide, sources linked to the WHO (World Health Organization) and the ILO (International Labour Organization) state that the working conditions of around 2/3 of the active population are below minimum quality standards, i.e. they represent a real risk to the health and physical integrity of individuals. Worldwide statistics show that there are around 157 million new cases of occupational diseases every year and 120 million accidents at work, 220,000 of which are fatal.

Index

Thanks

I would like to thank the publisher Novas Edigoes Academicas, without whom this book would not have been published. Veterinary science is a growing field these days, as more and more people have pets in their homes and treat them like family members. Our profession, which is emotionally and psychologically exhausting as well as physically demanding, has the aim of prolonging and supporting our four-legged friends. It entails numerous risks for professionals, through occupational accidents, animal bites or even attacks, and the psychological strain that has been proven to lead to numerous road accidents and depression.

I hope that this manuscript will help professionals to be more careful and attentive to small oversights that can sometimes be fatal or cause serious damage to health.

Thank you for this opportunity to evolve professionally!

Carla Patricia Costa

1. Introduce

The protection of workers' health is an indispensable element for the social and economic development of countries. The prevention of accidents, illnesses and injuries in the workplace must remain a priority. Much has been done to control work-related illnesses and accidents, especially over the last two decades (Oliveira and Andre, 2010).

Occupational safety and health conditions are regulated by numerous laws and regulations, whether general, sectoral or even relating to specific occupational risks. Currently, there are still high levels of accidents, which may reflect the poor or non-existent occupational risk prevention structures in many workplaces (Decree-Law No. 109/2000 of June 30). The need for safety, hygiene, prevention and training at work is, at the same time, a reflection on ourselves and our attitudes as priority players, increasingly dependent and demanding on work and everything it entails (Oliveira and Andre, 2010).

Safety, hygiene and health conditions in the Veterinary Medical Care Centre (CAMV) are the material foundation of any occupational risk prevention program and contribute to increasing competitiveness by reducing accidents (Decree-Law no. 441/91 of November 14, reformulated by Decree-Law no. 133/99) (Oliveira and Andre, 2010).

The permanent integration of Occupational Health and Safety Services (OHSHS) into the structure of the CAMV's allows them to better carry out certain activities that are very relevant to the prevention of occupational risks, such as the planning and coordination of internal control measures to be adopted in the workplace (Oliveira and Andre, 2010).

Several studies indicate that professionals spend most of their time in the workplace and are the biggest contributors to a country's economic and social development. In professional practice, workers are subject to risks that can deteriorate their state of health, making prevention a priority. This preventive attitude will lead to a reduction in illnesses and accidents at work, as well as in the degree and number of disabilities and absenteeism (Oliveira and Andre, 2010).

Knowledge of the relationship between work and health has been and will continue to be a necessary, but not sufficient, condition for organizing interventions to promote health and well-being in the workplace and prophylactic measures for injuries and illnesses related to work and the conditions in which it is carried out (WHO, 1981). Society and its political and economic structures need to take Occupational Health (OH) on as a priority objective, and build the necessary legal, technical-professional and material conditions to put it into practice. The current state of the organization and provision of OS care in Portugal is the result of a complex process in which political, social, economic and technical-scientific factors play a role. These factors, communicating with each other, created the objective and subjective conditions for the establishment, in the 1960s, of a legal model for occupational medicine services, which influenced the development of workers' health (Oliveira and Andre, 2010).

In particular, sharps accidents are an inherent risk of handling needles and other objects during the course of veterinary practice. Although a significant effort has been made to reduce these accidents in human medicine, a relatively superficial approach seems to be prevalent in veterinary medicine. A review of the scientific literature shows that OPC accidents are very common among veterinary surgeons (VMs), veterinary nurses (VNs) and veterinary assistants, and that serious adverse effects are also infrequent. Similarly, these risks can be passed on to the owners. Thus, clients can also be injured in clinics while restraining the animal or by prescribing injectable/fluid medication to be administered at home (Weese and Jack, 2008).

Despite the lack of potential transmission of blood-borne human pathogens, such as the AIDS virus (HIV) and hepatitis B and C viruses, there are a variety of potential problems in veterinary medicine. It is plausible that infections can occur through the inoculation of zoonotic pathogens such as certain arboviruses, organisms from the animal's skin *(Staphylococcus* spp., *Pseudomonas* spp.), organisms from biopsy aspiration *(Blastomyces, Pasteurella* spp., *Staphylococcus* spp., *Streptococcus* spp.) or modified live vaccines. Physical trauma can also occur and be significant, with serious needlesticks or lacerations resulting from poor animal restraint during administration or blood collection being of particular relevance. Accidental self-injection by the operator with substances such as vaccines, antimicrobials, chemotherapy, euthanasia products, and anesthetics also present potential risks ranging from local irritation to severe systemic reactions (Weese and Jack, 2008).

For reasons of occupational health, personal health and liability, veterinary practices should review the measures adopted to reduce the likelihood of OPC accidents and develop written protocols to prevent injuries. The aim of this study was therefore to assess the incidence of OPC accidents in TV and the association of these OPCs with potential risk factors. To carry out this study, questionnaires were drawn up for MVs and EVs to fill in. The questionnaires were designed taking into account various criteria/factors previously considered relevant in similar risk analyses.

2. History of occupational health

2.1. Ancient occupational health

The first known historical references to the negative relationship between work and health are described in the "Satire of the Professions", a document dating from 2360 to 2160 BC, which was attributed to a scribe from the Middle Eglpian Empire who, fearful that his son would not want to follow his career, reviewed all the main professions of the time and presented, without benevolence, testimonies from workers about the harmful effects of manual labor, including fatigue, poor hygiene and the threat of accidents at work. The first bibliographical references to occupational diseases date back to this period, compiled recently by Santos in 2004, namely reports of silicosis in gold and silver miners, as well as in the past in pyramid builders (Santos, 2004).

In ancient Greece, from the Homeric era to the Hellenistic era, there was an enormous evolution in working conditions, with the division of activities by sex, the proletarianization of the rural classes and the multiplication of professions in the urban setting with their progressive compartmentalization. The evolution and progress of work tools was also significant, and simple tools such as the lever, the wedge, the screw and the crane became known. The technique was still rudimentary, despite the notable development of some mechanisms such as the water mill and the wheel with buckets (Lefranc, 1988).

Knowledge of the negative effects on health of the activity of Greek craftsmen and miners from the 5th to 4th centuries BC underpins the value judgment attributed to Plato that there is a radical incompatibility between the practice of a mechanical profession and the duties of a citizen. For this philosopher and his contemporaries, "the beauty of the body and the beauty of the soul necessarily go hand in hand, an activity that makes the body shapeless makes the soul ugly, the obscurity of the workshop and the filth of the body produce counterfeit souls that have no sense of freedom, subject to another and interested only in gain" (Lefranc, 1988).

According to Santos (2004), Hippocratic medicine, for philosophical and political reasons, neglected to practise medicine on workers, whether independent or slaves, and therefore ignored professional illnesses.

Due to the barbarian invasions of the Western Roman Empire (from the fourth to the ninth centuries), trade came to a standstill and industrial activity stagnated to such an extent that in the tenth century, the evolution of production throughout Europe reached its lowest point. However, it was in the 11th century that the center of gravity of industrial life shifted from the domains of the monasteries to the reborn cities. In these cities, industrial work reappears in artisanal form, each profession is made up of free citizens who tend to focus on the same street or neighborhood. The organizational models of the Roman *"collegium"* are partly taken over. The purpose of these associations was not only to provide mutual assistance but also to control production, working conditions and the quality of products. They were responsible for setting limits on working hours and weekly rest days (Santos, 2004).

Their structure is progressive, both in its internal organization and in its external influence, particularly in the sharing of power in the cities themselves. Their economic and political importance in the organization of European societies is recognized through formal statutes, such as the English craftsmen of 1563 and the Portuguese professional associations of the 15th and 16th centuries (Schilling, 1981).

With the resumption of economic and commercial development in the 15th and 16th centuries, the necessary conditions were created for the development of the old mining industry, particularly in central Europe. In this context, the aggravated living and working conditions of miners led to a progression of medical knowledge of the pathologies linked to this type of work, going beyond the level of general knowledge and becoming the object of specific and targeted study. Agricola and Paracelsus, doctors from the Swiss region, deepen their knowledge of the work-related pathologies prevalent in mining communities, namely silicosis and tuberculosis. The published works contributed to raising awareness of the health problems of miners, facilitating progress in their professional status (Lefranc, 1988; Santos, 2004).

Georgius Agricola (1499-1555), a doctor from the mining town of Joachimsthal in

Bohemia, published a 12-volume work entitled *RE METALLICA* in which he described the tools, instruments and methods of mining production, paying close attention to ventilation and the pumping of water from the bottom of the mine. He ends his work with a detailed description of the most common illnesses and accidents among miners, as well as ways of preventing them (Graga, 2004; Santos, 2004).

He described "asthma" among workers who worked in mines full of dust: "Some mines are so dry that they are entirely devoid of water and this makes the workers even drier, which is harmful. The dust, which is stirred up and released by excavation, penetrates the windpipe and lungs, and produces difficulty in breathing, a disease they call asthma" (Graga, 2004).

Agricola's description and explanation of lung diseases is still not very rigorous, but this doctor has the merit of proposing the ventilation of mines and the use of a cloth over miners' faces, in order to improve working conditions and prevent diseases (Graga, 2004).

Another important historical reference, already mentioned above, is the physician Paracelsus (1493-1541), whose first monograph on the occupational diseases of miners and metal smelters was published in 1567. His clinical observations of miners' lung diseases are essentially current, even though the etiological explanation is based on the theory of tartar deposition. Unlike Agricola, he did not value the correctness of working conditions, concluding that the diseases observed were the price to pay for progress (Schilling, 1981; Santos, 2004).

Paracelsus is best known today as the "Father of Toxicology" because of his observations on dose and response: "All substances are poisons, there is none that is not a poison. The correct doses differentiate a poison from a remedy" (Graga, 2004).

The manufacturing boom that accompanied the Italian Renaissance, diversified and intensified production, worsening the working conditions of many workers and craftsmen. The Italian doctor and professor of medicine from Padua, Bernardino Ramazzini (1633-1714), was responsible for the first systematic study of occupational diseases, not only investigating the relationship between work and illness, but also presenting proposals for preventing or correcting working conditions. In 1700, he published the book *"De Morbis Artificum Diatriba"*, in which he mentions around 50 occupational diseases linked to the most diverse industrial professions, among others (Graga, 2004).

For almost two centuries it was considered a landmark work of occupational medicine and hygiene, where it was reprinted twenty-four times and translated into the main European languages. One of the first translations was the French *"Traite des maladies des ouvriers"* in 1770. There is a modern translation into Portuguese, made in Brazil by the Portuguese physician Raimundo Estrela (Graga, 2004).

The methodology of the work focused on surveying workers and direct observation of workplaces. This advance in the knowledge of work-disease relations remained current until the English industrial revolution, which also led to a revolution in occupational medicine (Santos, 2004).

In 1775, Percivall Pott (1713-1788), an English physician, drew attention to cancer of the scrotum in chimney sweep workers, based on clinical data recorded through systematic observations and the increased frequency of this pathology in this group of workers (Santos, 2004).

In 1784, Thomas Percival (1740-1804) was commissioned to study a typhus epidemic in the Manchester textile mills. In his report, he attributed the seriousness of the infection to long working hours and the accumulation of large numbers of workers in the same workplace. He advocated shorter working hours, a ban on night work and educational opportunities for workers, particularly children. Later, in 1795, Percival and his collaborators voluntarily took over the supervision of textile factories (Santos, 2004).

In 1832, the first English book on occupational diseases was published, entitled "The effects of the principal Arts, Trades and Professions and of civic states and habits of living, on health and longevity, with suggestion for the removal of many of the agents which produce disease and shorten the duration of life" by Leeds physician Charles Turner Thackrah (1795-1833). In this study, Thackrah and his collaborators describe the most frequent health problems in different types of employment, based on careful inspections of workers and interviews with employers, foremen and enlightened workers (Graga, 2004; Santos, 2004).

2.2. Modern occupational health

The intervention of occupational medicine in occupational health is, in the first place, linked to the progress and evolution of knowledge of occupational risks, having contributed significantly to public awareness of the physical, intellectual and moral misery resulting from the poor conditions in which men's work has been carried out over time (Schilling, 1981; Cassou et al., 1985; Santos, 2004).

In the twentieth century, international organizations such as the ILO and the WHO took on a dynamic role in the area of workers' health, promoting OS and making significant political and legislative progress since World War II, particularly in industrialized countries. The ILO is one of the oldest United Nations agencies, created after World War I and integrated into the League of Nations. After the Second World War, the ILO became part of the United Nations and, together with the WHO, has developed a number of proposals and guidelines of a general nature, influencing national laws and practices in many countries (Santos, 2004).

The ILO has the particular characteristic of being a tripartite body with representation from governments, employers and workers and its functions include improving working conditions by producing standards and international guidelines to be voluntarily signed by member states (Santos, 2004).

In theory, the ILO's influence is enormous since it has produced a vast set of directives and standards on occupational safety, hygiene and the organization of occupational health services that have promoted the development of OS laws and practice worldwide. In concrete terms, the impact of the ILO's standardization activity is not always so visible because the implementation of its guidelines on the ground faces numerous obstacles of a political and technical nature and a lack of qualified human resources (Dinman, 1987).

Recognizing the multiple repercussions of work on workers' health and well-being is based on up-to-date concepts of work and health and on the essential recognition of workers' participation in the process of producing knowledge in OS. The valorization of workers' and producers' health is the result of a contradictory historical evolution in which multiple factors intervene of a cultural, social and political nature that underlie the history of work and workers (Elling, 1986; Lefranc, 1988).

Therefore, in order to understand the current reality of the relationship between work and health and, in particular, to understand the rationale behind implicit and explicit policies on workers' health, it is necessary to know the historical past in order to identify the factors that have positively or negatively influenced the development of occupational health (Schilling, 1981; Elling, 1986; Santos, 1990).

Progress in the (philosophical and social) valorization of work, awareness of occupational risks and concrete intervention by actors in the world of work complete the interactive social system that promotes the political conditions for government intervention in the development of workers' health. The political and legislative edifice is then made up of policy instruments, plans and programs, norms and other legal documents, which, in continuous construction, shape the organization and provision of occupational health care at each historical moment (Emmett, 1997; Navarro, 1998).

According to the WHO, human beings are at the center of sustainable development, and OS is a basic constituent of the social and health dimension of that same development, understood, according to the Rio Declaration, as a strategy to meet the present needs of the world's population without causing negative effects on health and the environment, without depleting or endangering the resource base and without compromising the ability of future generations to meet their needs (WHO, 1995).

Policies and practices geared towards workers' health are thus the result of multiple influences and dimensions and, in a historical context, can be organized into three major phases of development, essentially following the author's essay on the evolution of the professional status of doctors and Matikaine and Rantanen's scheme, cited by Graga (2002), for the evolution of OHS in Europe: the Proto-Occupational Medicine phase from antiquity until the Second World War; the Classical Occupational Medicine phase from the Second World War until the 1980s and finally, the New Occupational Health phase from the latter date and still ongoing (Santos, 1990; Mendes and Dias, 1991; Emmett, 1997; Graga, 2002).

3. Evolution of labor protection legislation

3.1. Historical perspectives in an international context

It was through the influence of social reformers, philanthropic bosses, liberal politicians, philosophers and writers, humanist doctors, among others, that the defense and promotion of social and health protection for workers began through public activity and, consequently, the intervention of political power through legislation (Schilling, 1981; Graga, 2002).

The first labor legislation related to workers' health was known as the Morals and Apprentices Act of 1802. This was a decision by the English Parliament in response to a proposal put forward by the distinguished industrialist Sir Robert Peel, who followed up on field studies by the Manchester doctor Thomas Percival. This law began a long process of political intervention in regulating working conditions and supervising the negative effects of work-related health (Schilling, 1981; Santos, 2004).

The normative edifice was built through successive laws based on medical and social knowledge which essentially tended to reduce daily and weekly working hours, limit the age at which children and women could be recruited for industrial work, first in the cotton industry and then in the mines, metallurgical and chemical industries (Schilling, 1981; Duclos, 1984).

In 1833 the Factory Law was published, the first law to have any effectiveness, because it appointed the first four factory inspectors in charge of its application, and called, in an innovative but limited way, for the participation of doctors who were given the task of certifying that minors were of the minimum age to work - 9 years old (Schilling, 1981). From this year onwards, the regulation of the working day for young people is structured as follows: a ban on employment for minors under 9 years of age; a limit of 8 hours a day (six days a week of work) for minors between 9 and 13 years of age; a limit of 12 hours a day for adolescents between 13 and 18 years of age; a ban on night work for all minors and adolescents (Graga, 2002).

In 1841, the first law was published banning children under the age of 8 from working in factories with more than 20 workers and setting the working time limit at 8 hours for children aged 8 to 12 (Duclos, 1984).

In 1844, there was a further advance in the restriction of working hours, with a reduction to six and a half hours for children under the age of 13. Women under the age of 18 were included in the 12-hour maximum working day and were banned from working at night (Graga, 2002).

In 1847, the Ten Hours Law was published, culminating a long social and political battle. Its practical application to all industrial sectors took place throughout the second half of the 19th century. In France, following the industrialization process, the same legislative process also took place (Duclos, 1984; Graga, 2002).

By the end of the 19th century, all industrialized countries had adopted some kind of rules regulating working hours and the access of children, young people and women to industrial work. In the transition to the 20th century and before the First World War, with the publication of laws to compensate for damage caused by work, employers' liability for accidents at work and occupational diseases was finally legally recognized. In the case of England, the Accident Compensation Act dates from 1897 and the Occupational Diseases Compensation Act from 1906 (Graga, 2002).

There was little legislative progress in the period between the two Great Wars. The beginnings of occupational medicine are rooted in the company doctors voluntarily hired by some industrialists who were pioneers of the industrial revolution. With the 1833 Factory Act, the first compulsory medical expertise was created, assigning doctors the task of verifying the apparent age of children (9 years old) in order to enforce compliance with the age limit for admission to industrial work (Schilling, 1981; Graga, 2002).

Occupational pathology underwent significant changes with the industrial revolutions, moving from the pathology of each profession to a wide range of illnesses and afflictions of workers related to economic activities. In the new industrial working relationships, tuberculosis appears as a symbol of the difficult living conditions (Duclos, 1984).

The employed working population grew globally in the last 20 years of the 20th century and its distribution by sector of activity shows a growth in the tertiary sector at the expense essentially of the primary sector (Graga, 2002; Santos, 2004). In the twentieth century, international organizations such as the ILO and the WHO took on a dynamic role in the area of workers' health, promoting OS and making significant political and legislative progress since the Second World War, particularly in the industrialized countries (Santos, 2004).

3.2. Historical perspectives in a national context

The Portuguese reality highlights the inadequate and incongruous political-organizational model for providing occupational health care in the 1960s (Faria et al., 1985), which was replaced by the new legislation of 1994 and 1995 (Decree Law 26/94 and Law 7/95) and which supports a new formal HSEH structure that is far from corresponding to the reality of the evolution of productive forces, their organization and the health and well-being needs of workers (Santos, 1998; Graga, 1999).

The reformulation of Occupational Health policy, together with the reorganization of health services aimed at the working population, has been advocated by some authors and organizations since the beginning of the 1980s (Faria et al., 1985; Faria, 1988; Graga, 1999).

This need has recently become evident to all the social partners and the political authorities, which has triggered the current process of change, the first of which was the approval of the "Agreement on Safety, Hygiene and Health at Work" by the Permanent Social Concertation Council in July 1991, renewed by the "Agreement on Working Conditions, Hygiene and Safety at Work and Combating Accidents" of the Economic and Social Council in February 2001 (CPCS, 1991; CES, 2001).

The first impetus for the reform of occupational health services came with the publication of Decree-Law No. 1/85 of January 16, which adopted ILO Convention No. 155 on the safety and health of workers of 1981 (Decree-Law No. 1/1985).

At the end of the 1970s and the beginning of the 1980s, the trends in the economic development of the industrialized countries became clear. The growing economic resources coming mostly from the service sector and industry, and to a very limited extent from agriculture, make it possible to support social health, education, research and cultural services of an increasingly high standard (WHO, 1995).

This significant socio-economic development in industrialized countries has had an important impact on working conditions, health standards and occupational safety, changing the profile of the employed workforce (Mendes and Dias, 1991).

The introduction of new technologies, despite contributing to the improvement of general working conditions, ends up creating new health risks, almost always linked to components of the organization and the type of work itself (Mendes and Dias, 1991; WHO, 1995).

The commitment at national level to a new OS policy, made in the form of a law, did not have an immediate impact on the normative and organizational construction of the occupational medicine services that had been in place since the 1970s. It was to last until the first half of the 1990s, so much so that Faria, in 1994, noted that "the progress made in occupational medicine was slow and scarce, so that problems and trends persist which show resistance to change and an inability to learn from the mistakes of the past" (Faria, 1994).

The Ministry of Health, by Ministerial Order of March 13, 1985, demonstrated its intention to continue the process of legislative renewal by setting up a working group to review and update the legislation on OS, at the proposal of the General Directorate of Health (DGS). In light of this decision, it is expressly stated that the legislation (Decree Law No. 47511 and Decree No. 47512, 1967) is out of step with the socio-economic and political situation in our country, and with legislation issued by international organizations such as the ILO, the European Economic Community (EEC) and the WHO. Specifically, it is argued that the percentage of the population covered has not changed significantly over the life of the law (Information No. 35/1985).

According to the DGS's assessment, the existing legislation, on the one hand, makes it difficult to adopt an integrated OS organizational model in the official health services and, on the other hand, agricultural, commercial and service companies are excluded. Small businesses have not been able to create inter-company services and the few common services that do exist are not within the scope of current legislation. There is no provision for the necessary human and other resources for official services. Only occupational physicians are considered to be OS technicians and there are no rules for training others, such as nurses, industrial hygienists and hygiene and safety technicians, or for providing basic training for public health and general clinical physicians. There is no definition of professional statutes beyond company occupational physicians (Information No. 35/1985).

The arrival of the 1990s brought a new perspective to the old legislative and organizational edifice of occupational health created in the 1960s. The specific conditions in the country and the influence of international organizations such as the European Union, the European Organization of the WHO and, in particular, the ILO, make it possible to admit a new advance in workers' health (Santos, 1998).

3.3. Current legal framework for safety, hygiene and health at work in Portugal

Accidents that occur during the course of work and occupational illnesses are legally supported by national legislation, which defines the concepts of accidents in the course of work and the respective compensation for damages (Arrabago, 2008).

In 1991, all the social partners signed the specific agreement on SSHST at the Permanent Social Concertation Council and published its legal framework (D.L. n.° 441/91, of November 14), which refers to later regulations on various aspects such as the organization of care services, training of workers and their participation (CPCS, 1991; Decreto Lei n.° 441, 1991).

The political justification for this agreement lays down broad general or strategic objectives of a dual nature, aimed at companies and workers. The new HSE policy must, on the one hand, take account of changes in the business fabric and contribute to the objectives of modernizing the economy by increasing the competitiveness of companies and, on the other, ensure the improvement of workers' working and living conditions, satisfying their professional objectives and guaranteeing their well-being and social progress (CPCS, 1991).

The new OS policy is based on arguments that directly link improving safety, hygiene and health conditions in the workplace to stimulating creativity and motivating workers, developing skills and experience, increasing physical and psychological well-being and easing individual, family and group tensions. Therefore, working in safe and healthy conditions leads to a reduction in accidents and occupational illnesses and consequently to a reduction in direct and indirect losses for the company and occupational injuries. On the other hand, improving working conditions and valuing human resources helps to retain skilled labor and establishes a harmonious growth relationship between working conditions and competitiveness (CPCS, 1991).

Decree-Law 100/97 of September 13th is a framework law that approves the legal regime for accidents at work and occupational diseases and covers all workers on behalf of others, known as dependent workers (Arrabago, 2008).

On May 11, Decree-Law no. 159/99 was published, which, in accordance with Decree-Law no. 100/97, made it compulsory for self-employed workers to have insurance to guarantee the benefits provided (Airabaco, 2008).

Subsequently, due to the need to clarify the legal regime for accidents at work and occupational illnesses in the Public Administration, Decree-Law no. 503/99 of November 20th was published, establishing the legal regime for accidents occurring in the service of the Public Administration, since the last publication was from 1965 and was completely outdated and out of step with the new requirements. According to Decree-Law no. 503/99, the concept of an accident at work is considered to be "An unintentional and unexpected event that occurs at the place and time of work. An accident that occurs in the workplace and directly or indirectly produces: bodily injury, functional disturbance, illness and causes death, or a reduction in working or earning capacity" (Arrabaco, 2008).

In recent years, new laws have been created, with the publication of Law No. 99/2003 of August 27 approving the Labor Code and Law No. 35/2004 of July 29 regulating the Labor Code, which defines the regime to be applied to workers under employment contracts (Arrabaco, 2008).

3.4. Historical perspectives on American legislation

The progression of Occupational Health and Safety (OHS) in the United States took place during the Progressive Era, from the 1890s to the 1920s. Labor unions did much to influence improvements in occupational health and safety by influencing legislation. In 1914, studies in New York and Ohio revealed unhealthy working conditions causing diseases such as tuberculosis, which led to the abolition of sweatshops. Professional organizations were created such as the American Society of Safety Engineers, 1911; the National Safety Council, 1913; and the American Industrial Hygiene Association, 1939.

Once the Great Depression was over, in 1930, through President Roosevelt, the government approved labor standards set by the unions. A period of industrial growth began, as some of the gains of the last years before World War II were lost due to the need to maximize the production of artillery and war materials. From this moment on, new laws were created that have promoted improvements in occupational safety and health to this day (Abrams, 1994).

The Health and Safety Act, signed by President Richard M. Nixon on December 29, 1970, created both the National Institute for Occupational Safety and Health *(NIOSH)* and the Occupational Safety and Health *Administration* (OSHA) (CDC, 1999).

NIOSH was established to help ensure safe and healthy working conditions by providing research, information, education and training in occupational safety and health. NIOSH provides national and global leadership to prevent work-related illness, injury, disability and death by collecting information and conducting scientific research (CDC, 1999).

OSHA's main objective is to ensure that employers provide employees with an environment free from recognized hazards, such as exposure to toxic chemicals, excessive noise levels, mechanical hazards, heat or cold stress, or unhealthy conditions in their potential biological hazard (www.osha.gov).

Currently in the United States, the constant concern over sharps accidents has generated intense legislative activity to protect workers in the workplace from SO. Employees are obliged to conduct themselves in a cautious manner in order to avoid injury, however, statutes universally oblige employers to provide a safe working environment (Weese and Jack, 2008).

3.5. Legislation in a veterinary context

In addition to applying the general principles for promoting safety, hygiene and health at work, adopted by Decree-Law 441/91, of November 14, the rules for protecting workers from the risks of exposure to biological agents at work were established. This law transposes into national law Council Directives 90/679/EEC, of November 26, and 93/88/EEC, of October 12, and Commission Directive 95/30/EC, of June 30, 1995 (DL 84/97).

Workers can be exposed to biological agents that pose risks to their health in many activities, including veterinary clinics, research laboratories, hospital services, clinical and diagnostic laboratories, slaughterhouses, waste collection and treatment and in various branches of industry (DL 84/97).

Decree-Law 84/97 focuses on protecting workers, first and foremost by assessing the risks of exposure to biological agents, in order to identify the agents causing the risk, the possibility of their spread in the community and the time of actual or potential exposure of workers. At the same time, risk assessment has made it possible to formulate guidelines for the application of measures to protect workers from dangerous biological agents, as well as agents whose dangerousness has not yet been defined (DL 84/97).

Therefore, once the biological agents causing the risk have been identified, the owner of the VAM must avoid using these agents, whenever the nature of the work allows it. If this is not technically feasible, the owner of the CAMV must reduce the risk of exposure to the level that is technically possible to adequately protect workers, as stated in decree-law 84/97.

The risk assessment will also allow the owner of the VAM to subject workers to health checks in order to monitor the evolution of their state of health and, if necessary, adopt the appropriate preventive measures. This assessment should be reviewed annually in those VAMs where the usual casuistry suggests a greater risk of exposure of MVs and EVs to dangerous biological agents, namely when agents with a higher degree of risk are used, special protection measures should be applied to reduce the risk of infection. The prevention of occupational risks also depends, to a high degree, on MV's and EV's carrying out their work with behavior appropriate to the safety requirements imposed by the biological agents present. Training and informing workers about the precautions to be taken in activities where biological agents are used is therefore extremely important (Decree-Law 84/97).

3.5.1. Classification of biological agents in the light of applicable legislation

Biological agents that can cause infection in CAMV workers are classified according to their level of infectious risk into 4 groups. A group 1 biological agent has a low probability of causing human illness. The biological agent in group 2, on the other hand, can cause human illness and is a danger to CAMV workers, but is unlikely to spread in the community and for which there are, as a rule, effective means of prophylaxis or treatment. Group 3 then includes biological agents that can cause serious illness in humans and pose a serious risk to CAMV workers, and are likely to spread in the community, even if there are effective means of prophylaxis or treatment. Finally, group 4 includes agents that cause serious human illness and pose a serious risk to workers, and which are likely to spread widely and for which there are generally no effective means of prophylaxis or treatment (DL 84/97).

In veterinary activities likely to present a risk of exposure to biological agents, the owner of the CAMV must carry out a risk assessment by determining the nature and group of the biological agent, as well as the length of time workers are exposed to it (DL 84/97).

The legislation stipulates that the risk assessment must take into account all available information, namely the classification of biological agents that present or may present a risk to human health, the additional risk biological agents may pose to MVs and EVs whose sensitivity may be affected, namely by previous illness, medication, immune deficiency, pregnancy or breastfeeding. It should also take into account the DGS recommendations on measures to control biological agents harmful to workers' health and existing technical information on diseases related to the nature of the work. Potential allergic or toxic effects resulting from the work and knowledge of a worker's illness that is directly related to their work should also be taken into account, as they are no less important (DL 84/97).

In order to update the possible discovery of emerging agents or agents with altered virulence, the risk assessment must be repeated periodically and also if there is a change in working conditions that could affect the exposure of workers to biological agents (DL 84/97).

3.5.2. Reducing the risks of exposure to biological agents

The risk of exposure must be reduced to as low a level as is technically possible in order to adequately protect the safety and health of VMs and EVs. To this end, the applicable legislation (DL 84/97) states that the number of MVs and EVs exposed or likely to be exposed to the biological agent should be limited to a minimum. Work processes and technical control measures must also be modified to avoid or minimize the spread of biological agents in the CAMV (DL 84/97).

Collective and individual protection measures must be put in place if exposure cannot be avoided by other means, as well as hygiene measures compatible with the objectives of preventing or reducing the accidental transfer or spread of a biological agent outside the workplace. It is compulsory to use signs indicating biological hazards and other appropriate signs, in accordance with the safety signs in force.

Action plans must be drawn up in the event of accidents involving biological agents and the presence of biological agents used at work outside the primary physical confinement must be checked whenever necessary and technically possible (DL 84/97).

The means of collecting, storing and disposing of waste after treatment must be appropriate, including the use of safe and identifiable containers whenever necessary. Finally, work procedures must be used that allow biological agents to be handled and transported without risk (DL 84/97).

3.5.3. Health surveillance of CAMV workers exposed to biological agents

The owner of the CAMV must ensure adequate surveillance of workers for whom the results of the assessment reveal the existence of risks to their safety or health, through health examinations on admission, periodically and occasionally. Prior to exposure to biological agents, MVs and EVs must undergo a health examination, and it is up to the occupational physician to determine the frequency of subsequent examinations, taking into account the risk assessment and the provisions of paragraphs 2 and 4 of article 16 of Decree-Law no. 26/94, of February 1 (DL 84/97).

Monitoring the health of CAMV workers must allow for the application of individual health measures and the principles and practices of occupational medicine, in accordance with the latest knowledge, and include the recording of the worker's clinical and professional history, the individual assessment of the worker's state of health, maintaining biological surveillance, whenever necessary; screening for early and reversible effects (DL84/97).

In order to guarantee the improvement of biological safety in the workplace, the occupational physician or the entity responsible for monitoring the health of CAMV workers must propose to the owner of the CAMV the preventive or protective measures to be taken for each worker. Occasionally, if a worker suffers from an infection or other illness that may have been caused by exposure to biological agents in the workplace, the occupational physician or the entity responsible for monitoring workers' health must propose that all workers subject to the same exposure have their state of health assessed, in which case the assessment of exposure risks must be repeated (DL 84/97).

The owner of the CAMV must also ensure that workers are given information and advice on the health monitoring they can undergo after the risk exposure has ended (DL 84/97).

3.5.4. Hygiene and personal protection measures applicable in the CAMV

According to Decree-Law 84/97, in veterinary activities where biological agents are used that pose a risk to the safety or health of workers, the owner of the CAMV must prevent the MV or EV from smoking, eating or drinking in work areas where there is a risk of contamination by biological agents. They must also provide the worker with suitable protective clothing and ensure that all protective equipment is stored in an appropriate place, checked and cleaned, if possible before and obligatorily after each use, and repaired or replaced if it is defective or damaged. Procedures must also be defined for the collection, handling and treatment of samples of animal origin in order to minimize the risk of exposure to potential agents present in the sampled matrix.

MVP workers must be provided with adequate sanitary and changing facilities for their personal hygiene, as well as ensuring that eye drops and skin antiseptics are available in appropriate places, when justified. MV's or EV's must immediately report any accident or incident involving the handling of biological agents to the person responsible for the work or the person responsible for safety and health in the workplace (DL 84/97).

Before leaving the workplace, workers must remove any work clothes and personal protective equipment that may be contaminated by biological agents and store them in separate rooms created for this purpose. The owner of the CAMV must ensure that the clothing and personal protective equipment are decontaminated, cleaned and, if necessary, destroyed (DL 84/97).

3.5.5. Measures applicable exclusively to veterinary establishments

Veterinary establishments must take appropriate measures to protect the safety and health of workers. Risk assessment in these establishments must also take into account the likelihood of the presence of biological agents in animal patients and in samples and waste materials from them, and the risk inherent in the nature of the professional activities. The danger posed by biological agents present or likely to be present in animal patients and in samples and waste materials from them must also be taken into account (DL 84/97).

The aforementioned measures must include, in particular, the specification of appropriate decontamination and disinfection processes, the application of processes that guarantee the safety of workers when handling, transporting and disposing of contaminated waste. Finally, containment measures must be applied to isolation units where animals are infected or suspected of being infected by group 3 or 4 biological agents (DL 84/97).

The owner of the CAMV must provide workers with written instructions in the workplace and, if necessary, display posters on the procedures to be followed in the event of an accident or serious incident resulting from the handling of biological agents or the handling of a group 4 biological agent (DL 84/97).

3.5.6. Physical hazards in the veterinary context

Although significant effort has been put into reducing OPC accidents in human medicine, a relatively weak approach seems to be prevalent in veterinary medicine. OPC accidents are an inherent risk of handling needles and other materials during the course of veterinary practice. It seems that injuries caused by OPCs are very common among veterinarians and also their animal clients, with serious injuries sometimes occurring during the restraint of the animal and also during the administration of injectable drugs (Weese and Jack, 2008).

There are a number of risk factors in veterinary practice that can cause traumatic injuries. The circumstances of the examination or the treatment instituted can upset the animal, requiring the intervention of MV's or EV's to physically restrain animals. Many of the animals being treated are large and heavy, or may be capable of biting, kicking or scratching in response to handling (Fritshi et al., 2006).

In addition, many veterinarians, especially those who work with farm animals, spend a large part of their lives driving, mostly on secondary roads, in order to see and treat patients. Some of this driving is done at night and/or when the veterinarian is tired, and these factors can increase the risk of road accidents (Fritshi et al., 2006).

Australian scientists have identified animal-related injuries, particularly to dogs and cats, as an important consequence of veterinary activity. Animal bites can result in cellulitis, abscesses, and more serious sequelae such as septicemia, arthritis, endocarditis, and central nervous system infections. In addition to exposure to zoonotic diseases and the resulting infection from bites and scratches, veterinarians can also develop reactions to allergens of occupational origin, such as dog or cat hair (Epp and Waldner, 2012).

Veterinary professionals should be aware of the lethal effects that bites can have and avoid undervaluing this type of accident. They should be alert to the possibility of serious infection and the appearance of unusual pathogens, which, if left untreated, can be fatal (Epp and Waldner, 2012).

Because of occupational health, personal health and liability issues, veterinary practices should review the measures adopted to reduce the likelihood of accidents with OPCs and develop written protocols in order to prevent injuries (Weese and Jack, 2008).

3.5.7. Accident prevention measures for OPCs

In 1981, McCormick and Maki were the first to describe the characteristics of

OPC accidents among healthcare workers and to recommend various prevention strategies, including educational programs, encouraging safety behaviors that include avoiding recapping needles and using better needle disposal systems (Rapparini and Reinhardt, 2010).

In 1987, the *Centers of Disease Control* (CDC) recommendations for universal prevention included a guide on preventing accidents with OPCs, focusing on care during handling and disposal (Rapparini and Reinhardt, 2010).

Several studies on the prevention of accidents with needles and other OPCs were published between 1987 and 1992, and focused on the development and placement of resistant OPC waste containers, with suitable locations for needle separation and the training of MVs and EVs on the risks of recapping, bending and breaking used needles (CDC, 2008; Rapparini and Reinhardt, 2010).

Since 1991, when OSHA first published the Bloodborne Pathogens Standard to protect healthcare workers from exposure to blood, the focus of regulatory and legislative activity has been on implementing a hierarchy of control measures. This has included paying greater attention to minimizing risks related to OPCs through the development and use of engineering controls (CDC, 2008; Rapparini and Reinhardt, 2010).

In 1998, OSHA published in the Federal Register a set of information on "engineering and work practice controls used to minimize the risk of occupational exposure to bloodborne pathogens due to percutaneous accidents with contaminated OPCs" (Rapparini and Reinhardt, 2010).

In November 1999, the CDC and NIOSH published a document, "NIOSH Alert: Preventing Needlestick Injuries in Healthcare Settings", which advises CAMV owners and their workers on strategies for preventing OPC accidents. This document is intended to help healthcare services in their efforts to implement programs to improve the safety of healthcare workers (Rapparini and Reinhardt, 2010).

By the end of 2001, 21 US states had established legislation to ensure the evaluation and implementation of safety devices to protect healthcare workers from accidents involving OPCs. In addition, the Needlestick Safety and Prevention Act, signed into federal law in the United States in November 2000, authorized the recent revision of the OSHA document (published in 2001) to more explicitly require the use of CLOs with safety mechanisms (Rapparini and Reinhardt, 2010).

The CDC has recently presented basic measures to reduce OPC accidents, including educating all CAMV staff and volunteers about waste treatment and avoiding needle sticks. The reuse of needles should be avoided unless absolutely necessary. If recapping is necessary, use the method of holding with one hand, and with the other hold the cap with a mechanical device such as a drip or use a device for recapping needles (CDC, 2013).

Likewise, after using needles, they should be immediately placed in approved sharps containers and convenient access to the containers should be ensured. These should be available in all areas where needles may be used. You should also avoid using temporary or unapproved sharps containers, as these can lead to serious injuries and accidents. Ideally, you should never attempt to remove any object from a sharps container and you should never fill sharps containers beyond the designated filling limit. The use of protective equipment such as retractable needles or hinged syringe caps should be considered for protection and to avoid occupational accidents, and staff should never be moved with an uncapped needle (CDC, 2013).

Finally, the owner of the CAMV must ensure that all employees report all needlestick accidents and record information about the circumstances (CDC, 2013).

4. Material and methods

4.1. Questionnaires

In order to carry out this study, questionnaires were drawn up to be filled in by MVs and EVs. The questionnaires were designed taking into account various criteria/factors previously considered relevant in similar risk analyses (Weese, 2009) with some adaptations, while maintaining the anonymity of the participant. Over the course of 6 months (December 2012 and May 2013), the questionnaires were distributed by post, filled in online using the Google tool (Google Drive) and also made available at the IX Montenegro Veterinary Congress, held on February 23 and 24, 2013 at Europarque in Santa Maria da Feira.

Several questions were included in the questionnaires in order to characterize the risks to which these professionals are potentially exposed. These questions include demographic factors (gender, age, weight and height), professional factors (years of experience, type of clinic, working hours, occurrence of needle sticks/scalpel cuts and their consequences, treatment for eliminating OPCs and occurrence of other accidents at work) and finally personal factors (visual acuity, predisposition to tension breaks, whether the worker is right- or left-handed).

These factors were analyzed in order to carry out a detailed characterization of the occurrences of accidents caused by OPCs in occupational accidents at the CAMV and their consequences for workers' health. The OPCs relevant to this study were needle sticks and scalpel cuts. "Needle stick" was defined as any accidental cut, abrasion or perforation of the dermis with a needle, alone or mounted on a syringe, in the context of work at the veterinary clinic or hospital in the previous six months. "Scalpel cut" was defined as any accidental cut or abrasion of the dermis with a scalpel blade, alone or mounted on a handle, in the context of work at the veterinary clinic or hospital in the previous six months.

For statistical purposes, the variables body mass index (BMI), years of experience, age, daily hours and weekly hours were categorized. BMI was categorized according to the guidelines established by the World Health Organization (WHO) and calculated as the ratio of the individual's weight (Kg) to the square of their height (m), classified as underweight (<18.5), normal weight (18.5-24.99), overweight (25-29.99), and obese (>30) (WHO, 2013). Years of experience were categorized as not experienced (up to 0.99 years), not very experienced (1 to 2 years), experienced (2.1 to 5 years) and very experienced (> 5 years). Hours per week were categorized as average hours (6 to 40 hours per week), heavy hours (41 to 50 hours per week) and very heavy hours (> 50 hours per week). Age was divided into the categories of 20 to 30 years, 31 to 40 years, 41 to 50 years and over 50 years. Daily working hours were divided into the categories of 1 to 8 hours/day, 8 to 12 hours/day, and more than 12 hours/day. Daily working hours were divided into the categories 1-16 hours/week, 17-40 hours/week and more than 40 hours/week.

4.2. Sample size calculation

The sample size for a prevalence survey with finite population correction (10% precision level) was calculated using methods described previously (Daniel, 1999; Mesquita et al., 2012). As no information is available on OPC accidents in either MVs or EVs, an estimated prevalence of 50% was assumed, thus producing the maximum possible sample size (Macfarlane, 1997). Official reports from Portugal indicate that in 2012 there were 4,202 veterinary doctors (www.omv.pt/ordem/estatisticas/) and 180 veterinary nurses (AEVP, 2012). To anticipate non-response or lack of data, the sample size was over-represented by 5%. According to the sample size calculation, at least 353 VMs and 96 VNs would have to be included in this study.

4.3. Statistical analysis

Univariate and multivariate logistic regression analyses were carried out and the crude odds ratio (cOR) and adjusted odds ratio (aOR) were calculated to assess the associations between the variables included in the risk analysis and the occurrence of accidents involving OPCs in CAMVs. In order to achieve greater sample representativeness, the logistic regression analyses were carried out taking into account the population of CAMV workers, not distinguishing between EVs and MVs. P-values of less than 0.05 were considered statistically significant. All the analyses were carried out using GraphPad Prism ver. Software 5.01 (GraphPad Software, San Diego, CA) and the Epicalc package in the R software (R 2.15.1) (R Development Core Team, 2012).

5. Results

A total of 206 questionnaires were obtained, of which 96 belonged to EVs and 110 to MVs.

Of the 96 EV questionnaires, 82 (85.4%) came from women and 14 (14.6%) came from men. In the last 6 months of the study, 70 (72.9%) of the EVs had pricked themselves with needles and 26 (27.1%) had not pricked themselves with needles. There were a total of 243 needlestick accidents among IVs, of which 78 (32.2%) occurred when recapping; 48 (19.8%) when separating the needle from the syringe; 37 (15.2%) due to careless handling; 36 (14.8%) during blood collection; 20 (8.2%) with abandoned needles; 11 (4.5%) when suturing wounds or in a surgical context without an anaesthetized animal; 8 (3.3%) when passing needles from the hands of colleagues; 4 (1.6%) cases occurred when suturing wounds or in a surgical context with an anaesthetized animal and 1 (0.4%) was accidentally pricked by a needle found in garbage bags or clothes. Of the accidents recorded, 96 (39.5%) had pain; 32 (13.2%) had swelling as a result; 25 (10.3%) had bleeding and only 1 (0.4%) developed an allergic reaction. In total, there were 89 (36.6%) accidents in which there were no symptoms. With regard to the site of the bite, of the total number of accidents recorded, 125 (51.4%) occurred on the right hand and 118 (48.6%) on the left hand. Of the total number of needlestick accidents recorded, 94 (38.7%) were with needles containing antibiotics; 64 (26.3%) with animal blood; 60 (24.7%) with vaccines; 16 (6.6%) with anesthetics; 6 (2.5%) with sedatives and only 3 (1.2%) with euthanasia products.

No workers were exposed to the contents of syringes containing hormones or chemotherapy drugs as a result of being pricked. After using syringes with needles, 95 (99%) of the IVs put them in their own containers and only 1 (1%) used the garbage for disposal. Regarding the handling of needles fitted to syringes, 46 (47.9%) recap using both hands; 18 (18.8%) of EVs recap using one hand only; 16 (16.7%) use the proper structure for removing needles.

needles on the top of the needle containers; 8 (8.3%) recap with the aid of their mouth (biting the needle capsule); 6 (6.2%) place the needle and syringe directly in the needle container without recapping and 2 (2.1%) recap using drips/needle holders.

Regarding the occurrence of scalpel cuts in EVs in the last 6 months, 18 (18.8%) were cut with scalpel blades and 78 (81.2%) were not cut with scalpel blades. In all those who cut themselves with a scalpel blade, a total of 34 accidents were recorded, in 13 (38.2%) it occurred while separating the blade from the scalpel handle; in 8 (23.5%) it occurred while collecting surgical material after surgery; in 4 (11.8%) it occurred while processing surgical material for washing/sterilization; in 3 of them (8.9%) the cut occurred during surgery; In 3 of them (8.9%) the cut occurred with blades lost in garbage bags or clothing; in only 1 (2.9%) it occurred during support for surgery and in 1 (2.9%) it occurred with "abandoned" blades. With regard to post-cut symptoms with the scalpel blade, 11 (32.4%) did not have any symptoms; 10 (29.4%) had pain; 7 (20.6%) suffered bleeding and 6 (17.6%) of those who suffered cuts with the scalpel had swelling. None of the workers presented symptoms such as infection, fever or allergic reactions. Regarding the location of the cut, 17 (50%) cut themselves on the right hand and 17 (50%) on the left hand. With regard to the method EVs use to separate the scalpel handle/blade, 82 (85.5%) remove them using drips/needle holders; 12 (12.4%) remove the blade using their hands and only 2 (2.1%) remove it after washing and disinfecting.

Of the 110 questionnaires collected from VMs, 67 (61%) were from women and 43 (39%) from men. In the last 6 months of the study, 82 (75%) of the VMs had pricked themselves with needles and 28 (25%) had not. There were a total of 496 needle-stick accidents, of which 94 (18.9%) occurred during recapsulation; 89 (17.9%) occurred during suturing of wounds or in a surgical context without an anaesthetized animal; 83 (16.7%) occurred due to careless handling; 72 (14.5%) of the cases occurred during suturing of wounds or in a surgical context with an anaesthetized animal;

69 (13.9%) occurred when separating the needle from the syringe; 44 (8.9%) occurred during blood collection; 40 (8.2%) occurred with abandoned needles; only 2 (0.4%) occurred when passing needles from colleagues' hands and 3 (0.6%) occurred because

the needles were in garbage bags or clothes.

Of the needlestick accidents recorded, 202 (40.7%) had pain as a result; 69 (13.9%) had bleeding; 32 (6.5%) had swelling as a result and only 8 VMs (1.6%) had infection. There were no symptoms in 185 (73.3%) of the cases. With regard to the site of the bites suffered by the WLVs who suffered an accident, it was found that 298 (60.1%) were on the left hand, 184 (37.1%) on the right hand and only 14 (2.8%) on the legs. Of all the needlestick accidents, 163 (32.9%) were with needles containing antibiotics; 130 (26.2%) with animal blood; 79 (15.9%) with vaccines; 77 (15.4%) with anesthetics; 35 (7.1%) with sedatives; only 7 (1.4%) with euthanasia products and 5 (1.1%) with hormones. After using syringes with needles, 109 (99%) of the VMs put them in their own containers and only 1 (1%) threw the needles away. Regarding the handling of needles adapted to syringes, 45 (40.9%) recap using both hands; 23 (20.9%) put the needle and syringe directly into the needle container without recapping; 21 (19.1%) use the needle removal structure at the top of the needle containers; 12 (10.9%) recap with the aid of their mouth (biting the needle capsule) and 9 (8.2%) of the VMs recap with one hand.

With regard to the occurrence of scalpel cuts on VMs in the last 6 months, 30 (27.3%) were cut with scalpel blades and 80 (72.7%) were not cut with scalpel blades. Of those who cut themselves with a scalpel blade, a total of 60 accidents were recorded, with 23 (38.3%) occurring during surgery; 11 (18.3%) while separating the blade from the scalpel handle; 10 (16.7%) while supporting surgery; 7 (11.7%) while collecting surgical material after surgery; in only 2 workers (3.3%) it occurred during the processing of surgical material for washing/sterilization; in 2 (3.3%) it occurred during the opening of the wrapper containing the blade and in 1 (1.7%) it occurred with "abandoned" blades. 1 (1.7%) case occurred during the removal of stitches and 3 (5%) occurred during the removal of dressings.

Of the accidents recorded with the scalpel blade, 27 (45%) had pain; 20 (33.3%) had bleeding; 9 (15%) had swelling as a result of the accident; 3 (5%) had no symptoms whatsoever and only 1 (1.7%) had swelling. Regarding the location of the cut, 27 (45%) of the accidents occurred on the right hand and 33 (55%) on the left hand. With regard to the method used by the MVs to separate the scalpel cable-lamina, 90 (81.8%) removed it using drips/needle holders; 17 (15.5%) removed it using their hands and 3 (2.7%) removed it after washing and disinfecting.

The univariate analysis of the risk factors for suffering a needle stick in the last 6 months (table 1, attached) showed that veterinary workers (VWs) with 1 to 2 years' experience were 4.69 times more likely to suffer needle sticks than VWs with less than a year's experience (cOR; 4.69; 95%CI: 1.01-21.84, $p=0.049$). It was also found that VTs who work mixed shifts are 2.33 times more likely to suffer needle sticks than VTs who only work day shifts (cOR; 2.33; 95%CI: 1.14-4.7, $p=0.021$).

With regard to the visual acuity variable, wearing contact lenses is a protective factor for suffering needle sticks, compared to the group that does not have full visual acuity (does not see 100%), nor wears glasses or contact lenses (cOR; 0.1; 95%CI: 0.01-0.97, $p=0.047$).

The univariate analysis of risk factors for being cut by a scalpel (table 2, attached) in the last 6 months showed that TVs working more than 50 hours a week were 3.47 times more likely to be cut by a scalpel than those working less than 40 hours a week (cOR; 3.47; 95%CI: 1.39.25, $p=0.013$). With regard to the visual acuity variable, wearing contact lenses is a protective factor against being cut by a scalpel, compared to the group that does not see 100%, nor wears glasses or contact lenses (cOR; 0.28; 95%CI: 0.09-0.87, $p=0.028$).

The multivariate analysis of risk factors for suffering a needle stick in the last 6 months showed that VTs who work mixed shifts are 3.28 times more likely to suffer needle sticks than VTs who only work day shifts (aOR; 3. 28; 95%CI: 1.34-8.00).28; 95%CI: 1.34-8.01, $p=0.009$).VTs who experience vertigo once a day are 2.42 times more likely to suffer from needle pricks than VTs who experience vertigo once a year (aOR; 2.42; 95%CI: 0.047.23, $p=0.021$). VTs who had vertigo once a month were 1.28 times more likely to suffer from needle sticks than VTs who only had vertigo once a year (aOR; 1.28; 95%CI: 0.01-5.71, $p=0.043$). With regard to the visual acuity variable, wearing contact lenses (aOR; 0.1; 95%CI: 0.01-1.3, $p=0.046$) as well as wearing glasses (aOR; 0.11; 95%CI: 0.01-1.26, $p=0.022$) are protective factors for suffering needle pricks, compared to the group that doesn't see 100%, nor wears glasses or contact lenses.

The multivariate analysis of risk factors for being cut by a scalpel in the last 6 months showed that being included in BMI category B is a protective factor compared to workers who belong to category A (aOR; 0.61; 95%CI: 0.09-4.03, $p=0.018$).

Given the similarity of the cOR and aOR values for each variable studied, we can conclude that there are no confounding variables in this model that could cause bias.

6. Discussion

Currently, sharps accidents still do not receive enough attention in veterinary medicine, because information about the zoonotic pathogens that can be present in animals, about the harmful potential of veterinary therapeutic drugs, and about the direct physical injuries that can result from these accidents is not recognized or transmitted. The aim of this study was therefore to assess the prevalence of OPC accidents in TVs and the association of these OPCs with potential risk factors. The prevalence assessment could only be carried out on veterinary nurses, as it was not possible to obtain the minimum sample for veterinary doctors.

A total of 206 questionnaires were obtained, 96 from EVs and 110 from MVs. A total of 149 (72.3%) questionnaires came from women and 57 (27.7%) from men. In the last 6 months of the study, 70 (72.9%) of the EVs and 82 (61%) of the VMs had been pricked by needles. This incidence of needle sticks in VMs is in line with a previous study by Wilkins and Bowman (1997) in which, of the 2532 interviewees, 1620 (64%) reported one or more needle sticks in the same period. In a total of 2663 accidents reported, the most frequently injected substances included vaccines, antibiotics, anesthetics and animal blood, which is in line with the findings of the present study. In the present study, the substances most frequently conveyed by needle sticks recorded in accidents in VMs were vaccines, antibiotics, anesthetic agents and animal blood.

Another study by Weese (2008) found that 64% of veterinarians reported one or more needle sticks during their professional career, with vaccines accounting for 50% of cases. Causes for medical treatment included allergic reactions to the injected agents, serious injuries and lacerations. According to Weese, 58% of people confirmed that they had been pricked with a needle that had been exposed to animal blood, 52% with antibiotics, 52% with vaccines, and 17% with anesthetic agents. Similar results were reported in another Australian study (Van and Fritshi, 2004), where 71% of veterinary technicians reported needlestick accidents. Two thirds of these technicians had needlestick accidents during the administration of injections containing substances including antibiotics (13%), euthanasia products (11%), sedatives (9%), vaccines (8%), and anesthetics (8%). These data are in line with our study regarding the contents of syringes, in which 163 (32.9%) of all the accidents involving VLs who pricked themselves with needles were with needles whose contents were antibiotics; 35 (7.1%) were pricked with sedatives; 79 (15.9%) with vaccines; 77 (15.4%) with anesthetic agents; only 7 (1.4%) were pricked with euthanasia products; 5 (1.1%) hormones and 130 (26.2%) with animal blood. Of the total number of needlestick accidents recorded among IVs, 94 (38.7%) were needlesticks with antibiotics in the syringe, similar to IVs; 6 (2.5%) were sedatives; 60 (24.7%) were vaccines; 16 (6.6%) were anesthetics; only 3 (1.2%) were euthanasia products; and 64 (26.3%) were animal blood.

While the consequences of most needlestick accidents are apparently minor, potentially serious ones can occur. In a previous study (Wilkins and Bowman, 1997) serious reactions were observed including severe local inflammation, abscess formation, joint infection, localized necrosis, skin erosion, local nerve damage, brucellosis, severe allergic reaction, psychedelic experience, spasm of the larynx and bronchi, and abortion. Anthelmintics, euthanasia agents, and anesthetics were most commonly associated with adverse effects.

Some of these more severe consequences can be seen in this study, where 32 (6.5%) of the needlestick accidents in VMs resulted in swelling and 8 VMs (1.6%) resulted in infection. Likewise, of the accidents recorded in IVs, 32 (13.2%) had swelling as a consequence and 1 (0.4%) developed an allergic reaction.

Long-term or serious complications have also been reported in other studies. According to Patterson et al. (1988), the accidental injection of a horse vaccine (contaminated with *Mycobacterium avium* subspecies *paratuberculosis)* into a finger resulted in the presence of a small nodule that persisted for 4 to 6 months, with painful inflammation for 2 years. Ashford et al. (2004) described needle stick accidents containing the brucellosis vaccine (RB51), with 27% of the people studied reporting adverse reactions including erythema, fever, chills, sweating, fatigue, myalgia and arthritis, causing long-term adverse reactions (> 6 months). Accidental injection with an oil-based bovine vaccine in an agricultural worker resulted in the amputation of a digit as it resulted in ischemic necrosis (O'Neill et al., 2005).

In another study produced by Wilkins & Bowman in 1997, there was a serious side effect produced by the accidental self-injection of a prostaglandin compound which resulted in a spontaneous abortion. This type of accident with serious repercussions raises awareness that occupational needle stick accidents can also pose a serious risk to human reproductive health.

In this study, univariate analysis showed that VTs with relatively little experience (1 to 2 years of work) were more likely to have suffered a CTO in the last 6 months than those with less than a year's experience (cOR; 4.69; 95%CI: 1.01-21.84, $p=0.049$). This is to be expected, since individuals with very little experience (< 0.99 years) may not yet have enough professional confidence to take less thoughtful and riskier actions; this may already be the case in the group of individuals with between 1 and 2 years' experience, who may act with excessive confidence.

Multivariate analysis showed that TVs who work mixed shifts are more likely to have suffered an OPC in the last 6 months (aOR; 3.28; 95%CI: 1.34-8.01, $p=0.009$) than those who work the day shift. This is to be expected and is the result of fatigue and changing schedules, which can lead to both physical and psychological exhaustion and potentially less reflective attitudes and decisions. This association has already been described by Wilkins and Bowman (1997). The univariate analysis showed that workers who work more hours per day are more likely to have suffered an OPC in the last 6 months (cOR; 3.47; 95%CI: 1.3-9.25, $p=0.013$). This may be the result of TV fatigue, which affects not only the physical level but also the psychological level, altering posture in the workplace and reasoning and decision-making. In an Australian study by Fritshi et al (2006) and later in Kerala by Pillai (2012), it was shown that with an increase in the number of hours worked, both daily and weekly, there is a greater predisposition to accidents and injuries, supporting the findings described here.

With regard to multivariate analysis, it was found that belonging to group B on the BMI scale is a protective factor (aOR; 0.61; 95%CI: 0.09-4.03, $p=0.018$) in relation to BMI group A. This can be explained by the fact that TVs with very low BMI (level A on the scale) don't have enough muscle power to produce effective animal restraint. In this sense, any restraint could be compromised by insufficient muscle power, possibly hindering manipulation and leading to sharps accidents.

Veterinarians are highly susceptible to work-related injuries and illnesses due to the nature of their work and the demands of dealing with animals. A study was carried out in 2012 by Pillai, whose objective was to analyze and evaluate physical work injuries and associated risk factors among veterinarians in Kerala, India. This study found that physical injuries are of various etiologies and estimated that 6% of veterinarians were bitten by dogs, 8% were scratched by dogs, 3% were bitten and scratched by cats, 22% suffered OPCs, and the rest had other unspecific injuries, clearly demonstrating the association with physical injury.

Although this study does not focus on accidents caused directly by animals, it has made it possible to carry out a preliminary characterization of the occurrences of accidents with a physical etiology at the CAMV and their consequences for TV health in Portugal. From an analysis of the results, it is important to highlight the high probability of accidents occurring and their seriousness, taking into account the possible health consequences. Although there was no significant frequency of infections or symptoms suggesting them (e.g. fever) as a consequence of sharps accidents, we cannot exclude the possibility of the occurrence of zoonoses via the hematogenous route which, although rare, can have fatal consequences.

From these accidents there is the potential for infections to occur from the inoculation of pathogens such as arboviruses, organisms from the animal's skin (Staphylococcus spp., *Pseudomonas* spp.), organisms from aspiration biopsy puncture *(Blastomyces, Pasteurella* spp., *Staphylococcus* spp., *Streptococcuss* pp.) or modified live vaccines. Physical trauma can be significant, especially with large-gauge needles or severe lacerations that result from circulating or poorly restrained animals during injection or blood sampling. The injection of substances such as vaccines, antibiotics, chemotherapy, euthanasia products, and anesthetics also pose potential risks ranging from local irritation to systemic reactions.

This study concludes that accidents involving OPCs are very common in CAMVs. Although there are no reports in the scientific literature of serious injuries and consequences of these accidents in Portuguese veterinary nurses and doctors, safety plans for handling and disposing of OPCs should be implemented in each veterinary center in order to mitigate the effects of OPCs. Although the subject is still underdeveloped in Portugal, there have already been studies carried out in other countries, the conclusions of which are beginning to cause concern. More studies should be carried out, as there is little information, especially in terms of risk analysis, both for the TV and for the pet owners themselves, who often end up using injectable treatments at home. There is therefore an urgent need to maximize safety by implementing accident prevention systems in each CAMV, in order to comply with current legislation.

7. Bibliographical references

Alvarado-Ramy F, Beltrami EM (2003). *New guidelines for occupational exposure to blood-borne viruses.* Cleveland Clinic Journal of Medicine. **Vol. 70(5)**:457-465.

Arrabago MFSR (2008). *Service accidents among health professionals: identification, representations and behaviors in the face of accidental microbiological exposure.* Master's dissertation in health communication. Universidade Aberta, Lisbon.

Ashford D, di Pietra J, Lingappa J, Woods C, Noll H, Neville B, WeyantR, Bragg SL, Spiegel RA, Tappero J, Perkins BA (2004). *Adverse events in humans associated with accidental exposure to the livestock brucellosis vaccine RB51.* Vaccine. **Vol. 22**:3435-3439.

Babcock H, Fraser V (2003). *Differences in percutaneous injury patterns in a multihospital system.* Infection Control and Hospital epidemiology. **Vol.24 (10)**: 731-736.

Cassou B, Huez D, Mouse M-L, Spitzer C, Touranchet A (1985). *Les risques du travail, pour ne pas perdre sa vie a la gagner.* Paris, La Decouverte,

Centers for Disease Control and Prevention (1997). *Evaluation of safety devices for preventing percutaneous injuries among health-care workers during phlebotomy procedures-Minneapolis-St.Paul, New York City, and San Francisco, 1993-1995.* Morbidity and Mortality Weekly Report . **Vol. 46 (2)** : 21-25.

Centers for Disease Control and Prevention (1999a). *Improvements in Workplace Safety : United States, 1900-1999.* Morbidity and Mortality Weekly Report. **Vol. 48(22)** :461-468.

Centers for Disease Control and Prevention (1999b). *Heat-Related Illnesses and Deaths: Missouri, 1998, and United States, 1979--1996.* Morbidity and Mortality Weekly Report. **Vol. 48(22)**:469-484.

Centers for Disease Control and Prevention (2008). *Workbook for designing, implementing, and evaluating a sharps injury prevention program.* USA, Department of Health & Human Services.

Cheng H-C, C-Y, Yen AMF-G, Huang C-F (2012). *Factors affecting occupational exposure to needlestick and sharp injuries among dentists in Taiwan: a nationwide survey.* Plos One. **Vol. 7(4)**: e34911.

Chongsuvivatwong V (2008). *Analysis epidemiological data using R and Epicalc.* Thailand, Epidemiology Unit Prince of Songkla University.

Conceigao C, McCarthy M (2011). *Public health research systems in the European Union.* Health Research Policy and Systems. **Vol.9**:38.

Permanent Council for Social Consertation - CPCS (1991). *Agreement on safety, hygiene and health at work.* Lisbon: Conselho Permanente de Consertagao Social.

Economic and Social Council - ESC (2001). *Agreement on working conditions, health and safety at work and combating accidents.* Lisbon: Economic and Social Council.

Constable PJ, Harrington JM (1982). *Risks of zoonoses in a veterinary service.* British Medical Journal. **Vol. 23(284)**:246-248.

Daniel WW (1999). *Biostatistics: A Foundation for Analysis in the Health Sciences. New York, John Wiley & Sons.*

Davis RG *(2008).HIV/AIDS education: Still an important issue for veterinarians. Public Health reports.* ***Vol.123 (3)****:266-75.*

Decree-Law No. 47 511/67 - "D.R", I Serie - A. 21 (25-1-67), 125-126.
Decree-Law No. 47 512/67 - "D.R", I Serie - A. 21 (25-1-67), 126-128.
Decree-Law No. 1/85- "D.R." I Serie - A. 13 (16-01-85), 110-122.
Decree-Law No. 441/91 - "D.R", I Serie - A. 262 (14-11-91), 5826-5833.
Decree-Law No. 26/94 - "D.R", I Serie - A. 26 (1-2-94), 480-486.
Decree-Law No. 7/95 - "D.R", I Serie - A. 75 (29-3-95),1710-1713.
Decree-Law No. 84/97- "D.R", I Serie - A, 89 (16-04-97), 1701-1709.
Decree-Law No. 100/97 - "D.R", I Serie - A. 212 (13-09-97), 4910-4917.
Decree-Law No. 503/99 - "D.R", I Serie - A. 271 (20-11-99), 8241 to 8256.

Dinman BD (1987). *Impact of the international labor organization on occupational health and safety laws and practice.* Journal of Occupational Medicine.**Vol.29(4)**:345- 352.

Doug H (1996). *Occupational health and safety in veterinary practice.* Canadian Veterinary Journal. **Vol. 37(10)**: 581-582.

D'Souza E, Barraclough R, Fishwick D, Curran A (2009). *Management of occupational health risks in small-animal veterinary practices. Occupational Medicine.* ***Vol.59****:316-322.*

Duclos D *(1984). La sante et le travail. Paris, La Decouverte.*

Elling RH *(1986). The struggle for workers' health: a study of six industrialized countries. New York, Baywood Publishing Company.*

Emmett EA (1997). *Occupational health and safety in national development: the case of Australia.* Scandinavian Journal of Work Environment and Health. **Vol. 23**: 324-333.

Epp T, Waldner C (2012a). *Occupational health hazards in veterinary medicine: zoonoses and other biological hazards.* Canadian Veterinary Journal. **Vol. 53**:144150.

Epp T, Waldner C (2012b). *Occupational health hazards in veterinary medicine: Physial, psychological and chemical hazards*. Canadian Veterinary Journal. **Vol.53**:151-157.

European Agency for Safety and Health at Work (2008).*Risk assessment and injuries needle stick (EFACTS 40),* consulted on 21-05-2013.
URL: https://osha.europa.eu/pt/publications/e-facts/efact40.

Faria M, Santos CS, Sales AA, Rosario MDP (1985). *Occupational health in Portugal: current situation, prospects for the future.* Lisbon: Caixa Nacional de Seguros de Doengas Profissionais.

Faria M (1994). *The practice of occupational medicine in Portugal: problems and trends.* In Congresso da Medicina do Trabalho, 3, Povoa de Varzim.

Fritschi L (2000). *Cancer in veterinarians.* Occupational Environment Medicine.**Vol. 57**:289-297.

Fritschi L, Day L, Shirangi A, Robertson I, Lucas M, Vizard A (2006). *Injury in Australian veterinarians.* London, Occupational Medicine. **Vol.56**:199-203.

Garcia-Alvarez L, Dawson S, Cookson B, Hawkey P(2012). *Working across the veterinary and human health sectors.* Journal of Antimicrobial Chemotherapy. **Vol.67**:

i37-49.

Gordon SS (1964). *Health hazards to health workers - a neglected area.* American Journal Public Health Nations Health. **Vol.54(6)**: 1001-1003.

Govind RP (2012). *Work related physical injuries and associated risk factors among veterinarians in Kerala.* Trivandrum, Achutha Menon Centre for Health Science Studies, Sree Chitra Tirunal Institute for Medical Sciences and Technology, Working.

Graga L (1999). *Promoting health in the workplace: the new occupational health?* Lisbon, Cadernos Avulso da Sociedade Portuguesa de Medicina do Trabalho. 1:7-96.

Graga L (2002). *History of Occupational Health and Safety in Europe.* In: Higiene, Seguranga, Saude e Prevengao de Acidentes de Trabalho (5ª Edigao). Lisbon, Verlag Dashofer.

Graga L (2004). *Health policies at work: a sociological survey of Portuguese companies.* PhD thesis. Lisbon, Universidade Nova de Lisboa.

Harvey JM (1999). *Analyzing Data with GraphPad Prism.* GraphPad Software Inc., San Diego CA.

Hunter D, Raffle A (1987). *Hunter's diseases of occupations* (6th edition). London, Hodder & Stoughton.

Ind JE, Jeffries DJ (1999). *Needlestick injury in clothing industry workers and the risks of blood-borne infection.* Occupational Medicine. **Vol. 49**: 47-49.

Information No. 35/85 Ministry of Health. Directorate-General for Primary Health Care . February 5: 1-4.

Kabuusu R, Keku E, Kiyini R, McCam T (2010). *Prevalence and patterns of self reported animal related injury among veterinarians in metropolitan Kampala. Journal Veterinary science. **Vol. 11(4)**: 363-365.*

Lefranc G (1988). *History of work and workers.* Lisbon. Europress.

Leggat PA, Smith DR, Speare R (2009). *Exposure rate of needlestick and sharps injuries among Australian veterinarians.* Journal of occupational Medicine and Toxicology. **4**:25

Lucas M, Day L, Shirangi A, Fritschi L (2009). *Significant injuries in Australian veterinarians and use of safety precautions.* London, Occupational Medicine. **59**:327-33.

Macfarlane SB (1997). *Conducting a Descriptive Survey: 2. Choosing a Sampling Strategy.* Tropical Doctor. **27**:14-21.

Makary MA, Al-Attar A, Holzmueller CG, Sexton JB, Syin D, Gilson M, Sulkowski MS, Pronovost PJ (2007). *Needlestick injuries among surgeons in training.* The New England Journal of Medicine. **Vol. 356(26)**:2693-9.

Mendes R, Dias EC (1991). *From occupational medicine to occupational health worker.* Revista de Saude Publica. ***Vol.* 25(5)**: 341-349.

Mesquita JR, Nobrega C, Vala H, Sousa SIV (2012). *Statistics in veterinary nursing research: what to know before starting the study.* The Veterinary Nurse. **Vol.3 (10)**: 594 - 598.

Naing L, Winn T, Rusli BN (2006). *Practical issues in calculating the sample size for prevalence studies.* Archives of Orofacial Sciences. **Vol.1**:9-14.

National Institute for Occupational Safety and Health- NIOSH (1999). *Preventing needlestick injuries in health care settings.* w.w.w.cdc.gov/niosh/2000- 108.html, consulted on 4/05/2013.

National Institute for Occupational Safety and Health- NIOSH (1999). *Preventing Needlestick injuries in health care settings.* w.w.cdc.gov/niosh/docs/2000-108.html, consulted on 4/05/2013.

National Institute for Occupational Safety and Health- NIOSH (2000). *What every worker should know: how to protect yourself from Needlestick injuries* . w.w.w.cdc.gov/niosh/docs/2000-135/, consulted on 4/05/2013.

Navarro V (1998). *A historical review (1965-1997) of studies on class, health and quality of life: a personal account.* International Journal of Health Services. **Vol. 28(3)**: 389-406.

Oliveira A, Andre S (2010). *Occupational health nursing.* Millenium. **Vol. 41**:115-122.

O'Neill J, Richards S, Ricketts D, Patterson M (2005). *The effects of injection of bovine vaccine into a human digit: A case report.* Environmental health: A global access science source. **Vol.4**:21.

Patterson C, LaVenture M, Hurley S, Davis J (1988). *Accidental self-inoculation with Mycobacterium paratuberculosis bacterin (Johne's bacterin) by veterinarians in Wisconsin.* Journal American Veterinary Medicine Association. **Vol. 192**:1197-1199.

Rapparini C, Reinhardt EL (2010). *Manual de implementagdo Programa de prevengdo de acidentes com materiais perfurocortantes em servigos de saŭde.* Sao Paulo, Fundacentro.

Rabinowitz P, Scotch M, Contri L (2009). *Human and animal sentinels for shared health risks.* Veterinaria Italiana. **Vol.45 (1)**: 23-24.

R Development Core Team (2012). *R: A language and environment for statistical computing.* Vienna, Austria , R Foundation for Statistical Computing.

Russi M, Butcha ., Swift M, Budnick L, Hodgson M, Berube D, Kelafant G (2009). *Guidance for occupational health services in Medical Centers.* Journal Occupational Environment Medicine. **Vol.51 (11)**:1e-18e.

Santos C (1990). *Technical-legal framework for the practice of occupational medicine: a critical analysis.* Jornal das Ciencias Medicas.**Vol.14 (7)**: 381-386.

Santos C (1998). *Innovative strategies in occupational health: the perspective of health centers.* Portuguese Journal of Public Health. **Vol. 16(1)**: 5-11.

Santos C (2004). *Development of occupational health in Portugal and the professional practice of occupational physicians.* National School of Public Health: New University of Lisbon.

Schilling R (1981). *Developments in occupational health.* In: Schilling R. Occupational health practice (2ª Edigao). London, Butterworth's: 3-25.

Sctoch M, Odofin L, Rabinowitz P (2009). *Linkages between animal and human health sentinela data.* Biomed Central veterinary research. **Vol. 5**:15.

Semmence A, Radwanski D (1984). *Occupational health and the general practitioner.* Journal of the Royal College of General Practitioners. **Vol. 34(265)**: 459-460.

Shiao J, Guo L, Mclaws ML (2002). *Estimation bloodborne pathogens to health care workers after a needlestick injury in taiwan.* American journal of infection control. **Vol. 30 (1).**

Steele JH (1973). *A Bookshelf on Veterinary public health.* American Journal Public Health. **Vol.63(4)**:291-311.

Stark KDC, Regule G, Hernandez J, Knopf L, Fuchs K, Morris RS, Davies P (2006). *Concepts for risk-based surveillance in the field of veterinary medicine and veterinary public health: review of current approaches.* Biomed Central Health Services Research. **Vol.6**.

Thompson RN, McNicholl BP (2010). *Needlestick and infection with horse vaccine.* British Medical Journal.

Van SE, Fritschi L (2004). *Occupational health risks in veterinary nursing: An exploratory study.* Australian Veterinary Journal. **Vol. 82**:346-350.

Weese JS, Peregrine AS, Armstrong (2002). *Occupational health and safety in small animal veterinary practice: Part I - nonparasitic zoonotic diseases.* Canadian Veterinary Journal. **Vol. 43 (8)**: 631-636.

Weese JS, Jack DC (2008). *Needlestick injuries in veterinary medicine.* Canadian Veterinary Journal. **Vol.49 (8)**:780-784.

Weese JS, Faires M (2009). *A survey of a needle handling practices and needlestick injuries in veterinary technicians.* Canadian Veterinary Journal. **Vol 50**:1278-1282.

Wicker S, Cinatl J, Berger A, Doerr HW, Gottschalk R, Robernau HF(2008). *Determination of risk of infection with blood-borne Pathogens following a needlestick* *injury in Hospital Workers.* Annals of Occupational *Hygiene.* **Vol.52 (7)**: 615-622.

Wilkins JR, Bowman ME_(1997). *Needlestick injuries among female veterinarians: frequency, syringe contents and side-effects.* Occupational Medicine. **Vol. 47**: 451457.

World Health Organization (WHO) (1995). *Global strategy on occupational health for all: the way to health at work.* Geneva, WHO library.

World Health Organization (WHO) (2009). *Global health risks: Mortality and burden of disease attributable to selected major risks.* Suiga, WHO library.

www.osha.gov/SLTC/bloodbornephatogens/index.htmlwww.cdc.gov/healthypets-
www.mte.gov.br_
www.riscobiologico.orgwww.msha.gov/REGS/ACT/ACTTC.HTM

ANNEXES

Table 1. Univariate and multivariate analysis of the risk of needle sticks in veterinary workers

Variables	Univariate		Multivariate	
	crude OR (95% CI)	p	adjusted OR (95% CI)	p
BMI				
A (<18,5)	**Ref**		**Ref**	
B (18,5-24,99)	0.28 (0.03,2.34)	0,241	0.31 (0.03,2.99)	0,31
C (25-29,99)	0.25 (0.03,2.32)	0,223	0.27 (0.03,2.96)	0,287
D(>30)	0.75 (0.04,14.58)	0,849	1.46 (0.06,34.51)	0,815
Weekly hours				
A (1 - 40h)	**Ref**		**Ref**	
B(41 - 50h)	1.54 (0.7,3.37)	0,284	1.5 (0.58,3.93)	0,405
C(> 50h)	2.16 (0.79,5.93)	0,135	1.27 (0.37,4.35)	0,024
Visual acuity				
He can't see 100% but he doesn't wear glasses or contact lenses	**Ref**		**Ref**	
Wears contact lenses	0.1 (0.01,0.97)	0,047	0.1 (0.01,1.3)	0,046
Wears glasses	0.21 (0.02,1.8)	0,153	0.11 (0.01,1.26)	0,022
See correctly	0.13 (0.02,1.04)	0,055	0.12 (0.01,1.2)	0,071
Years of experience				
A (up to 0.99)	**Ref**		**Ref**	
B (1 to 2)	4.69 (1.01,21.84)	0,049	4.51 (0.78,26.13)	0,093
C (2.1 to 5)	2.01 (0.77,5.26)	0,155	2.07 (0.66,6.42)	0,21
D (>5)	0.78 (0.33,1.88)	0,581	0.93 (0.34,2.54)	0,881
Working hours				
Daytime	**Ref**		**Ref**	
Evening	0 (0.Inf)	0,988	0 (0.Inf)	0,997
Mixed	2.33 (1.14,4.76)	0,021	3.28 (1.34,8.01)	0,009
Vertigo				
1 time per year	**Ref**		**Ref**	
1 time per month	0.25 (0.03,2.32)	0,223	1.28 (0.01,5.71)	0,043
1 time per week	0.75 (0.04,14.58)	0,849	0.64 (0.02,20.62)	0,992
Once a day	0.28 (0.03,2.34)	0,241	2.42 (0.04,7.23)	0,021
Never	0.52 (0.24,11.81)	0,532	0.44 (0.12,22.45)	0,688

BMI: body mass index; **Ref:** reference; **CI:** confidence interval; **OR:** odds ratio.

Table 2. Univariate and multivariate analysis of the risk of scalpel cuts in veterinary workers

Variables	Univariate		Multivariate	
	crude OR (95% CI)	p	adjusted OR (95% CI)	p
BMI				
A (<18,5)	**Ref**		**Ref**	
B (18,5-24,99)	0.79 (0.15,4.08)	0,779	0.61 (0.09,4.03)	0,018
C (25-29,99)	2.06 (0.36,11.91)	0,42	0.25 (0.33,15.23)	0,406
D(>30)	0 (0.Inf)	0,987	0 (0.Inf)	0,991
Weekly hours				
A (1 - 40h)	**Ref**		**Ref**	
B(41 - 50h)	1.69 (0.67,4.27)	0,265	1.8 (0.62,5.19)	0,28
C(> 50h)	3.47 (1.3,9.25)	0,013	3.33 (1,11.07)	0,05
Visual acuity				
He can't see 100% but he doesn't wear glasses or contact lenses	**Ref**		**Ref**	
Wears contact lenses	**0.2 (0.03,1.18)**	**0,075**	**0.31 (0.04,2.22)**	**0,246**
Wears glasses	**0.35 (0.1,1.25)**	**0,107**	**0.4 (0.09,1.67)**	**0,208**
See correctly	**0.28 (0.09,0.87)**	**0,028**	**0.42 (0.12,1.55)**	**0,195**
Years of experience				
A (up to 0.99)	**Ref**		**Ref**	
B (1 to 2)	2.08 (0.71,6.13)	0,183	1.52 (0.45,5.11)	0,498
C (2.1 to 5)	0.83 (0.29,2.36)	0,725	0.9951 (0.298,3.3231)	0,994
D (>5)	0.77 (0.25,2.36)	0,652	0.54 (0.15,1.9)	0,338
Working hours				
Daytime	**Ref**		**Ref**	
Evening	0 (0.Inf)	0,989	0 (0.Inf)	0,995
Mixed	1.23 (0.57,2.67)	0,601	0.67 (0.25,1.78)	0,422
Vertigo				
1 time per year	**Ref**		**Ref**	
1 time per month	0.62 (0.09,4.01)	0,611	1.13 (0.12,10.86)	0,917
1 time per week	1 (0.1342,7.4511)	1	1.92 (0.18,20.33)	0,588
Once a day	0 (0.Inf)	0,992	0 (0.Inf)	0,997
Never	0.43 (0.07,2.55)	0,356	0.58 (0.06,5.11)	0,621

BMI: body mass index; **Ref:** reference; **CI:** confidence interval; **OR:** odds ratio.

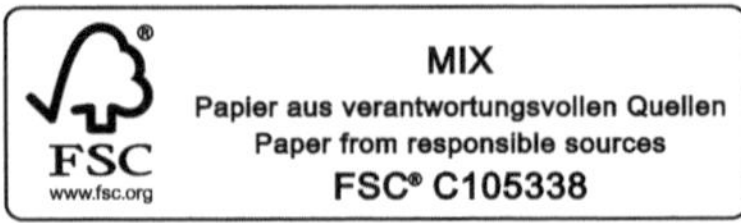

Printed by Books on Demand GmbH, Norderstedt / Germany